I am
worthy of
love and
respect.

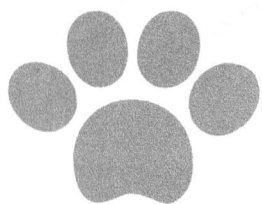

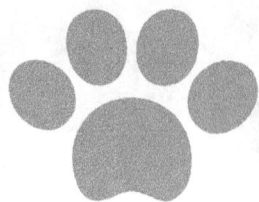

I love and accept myself unconditionally.

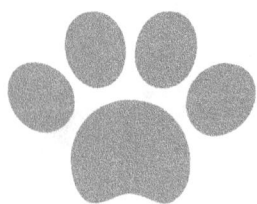

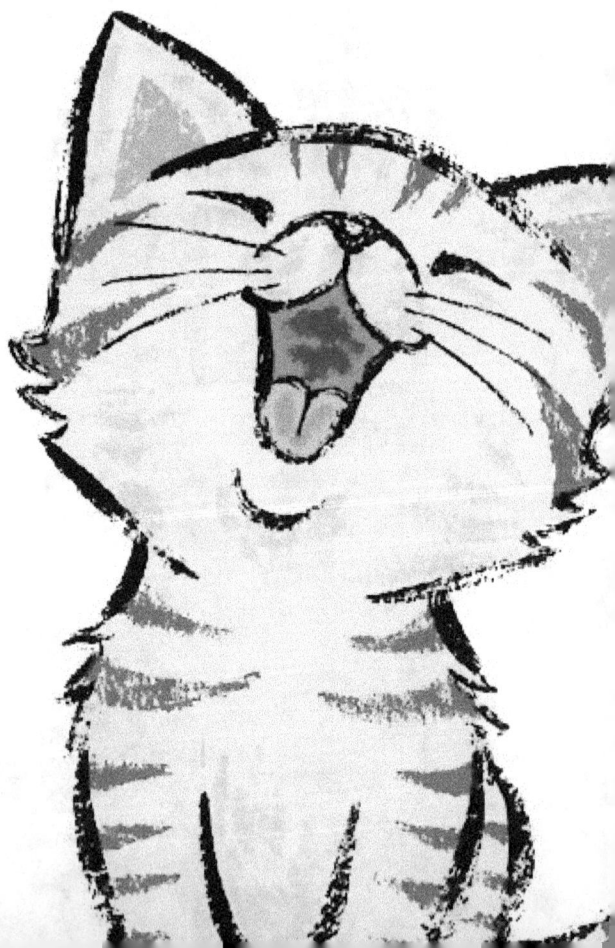

I am capable of achieving my goals and dreams.

I am confident in my abilities and intelligence.

I embrace my unique qualities and express myself authentically

I am strong and resilient in the face of challenges.

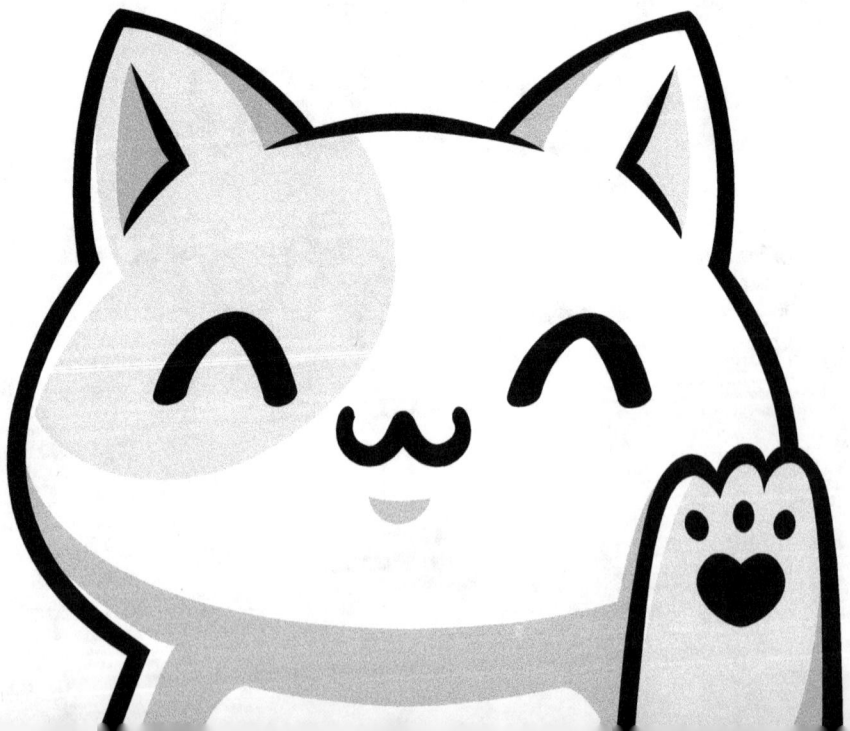

I deserve happiness and fulfillment in all aspects of life.

I am attractive inside and out, and I radiate positive energy.

I prioritize self-care and nurture my mind, body, and soul.

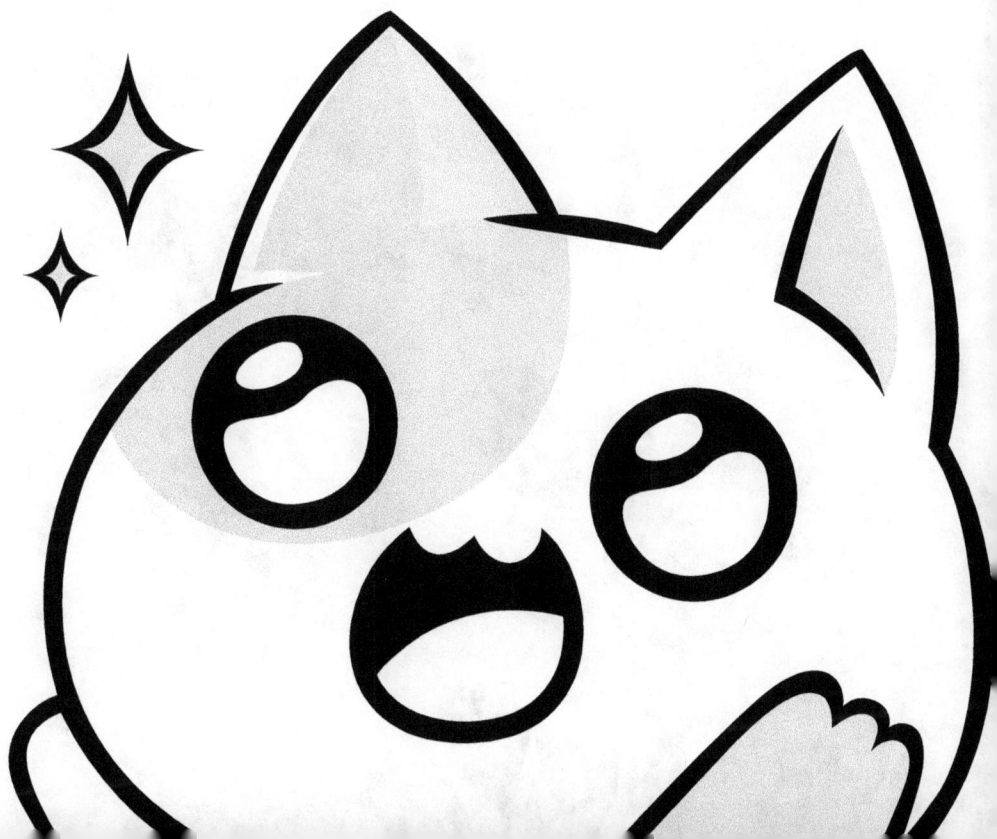

I am deserving of success and prosperity.

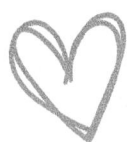

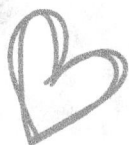

I am kind, compassionate, and understanding towards myself and others.

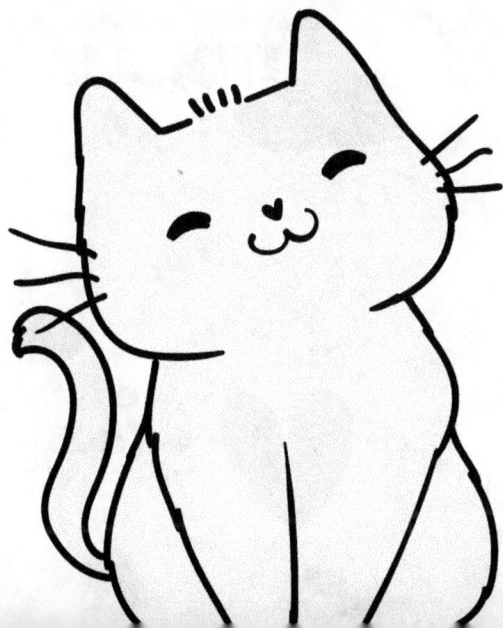

I am in control of my thoughts and emotions.

I forgive
myself
for past
mistakes
and focus
on
growth.

I am deserving of love, respect, and success

I am open to
receiving
love and
support
from others.

I am confident in expressing my needs and desires.

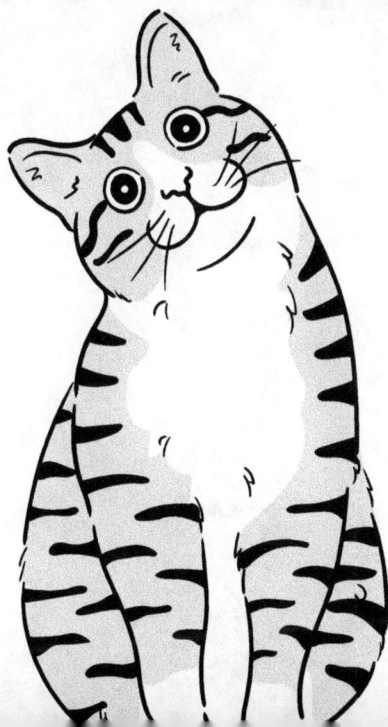

I trust my
intuition and
make wise
decisions.

I am
deserving of
love and
affection in
all my
relationships.

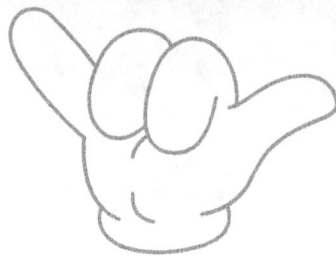

I embrace my uniqueness and celebrate my individuality.

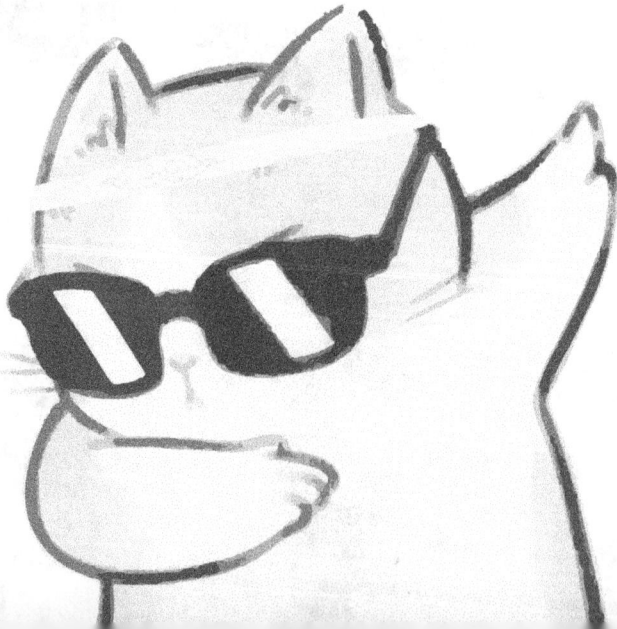

I am
constantly
growing and
evolving into a
better version
of myself.

I am
confident
and capable
in
everything
I do.

I am in tune with my emotions and handle them with grace.

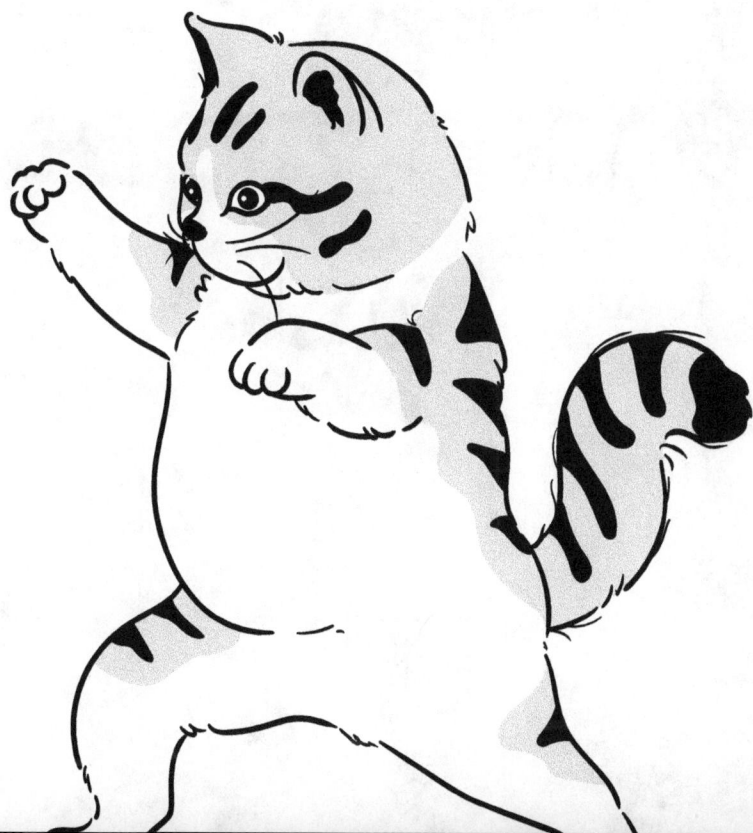

I am a positive influence on those around me.

I believe in my ability to overcome any obstacle that comes my way.

I love and accept myself just as I am.

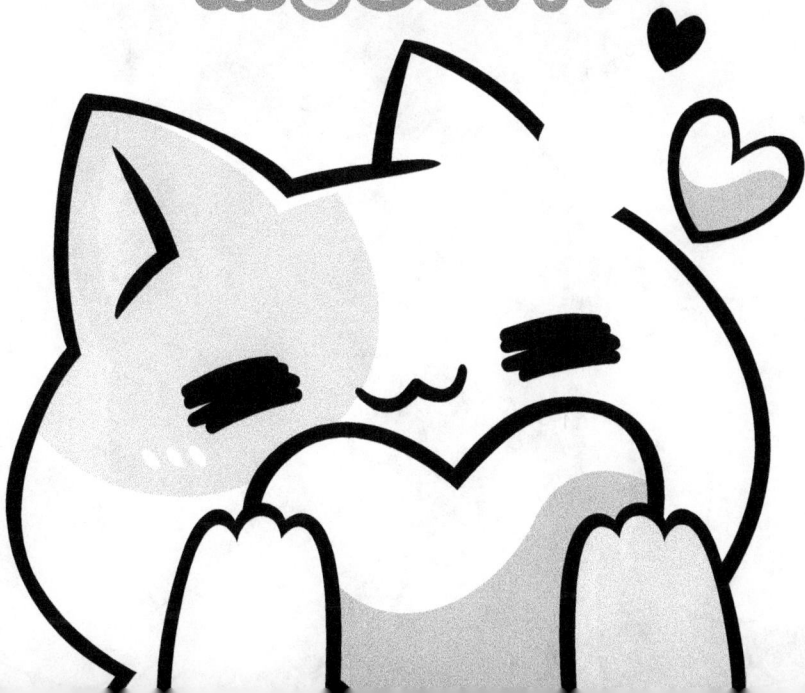

I am
beautiful
inside and
out, and I
radiate
confidence.

I am
capable of
achieving
my goals
and
aspirations.

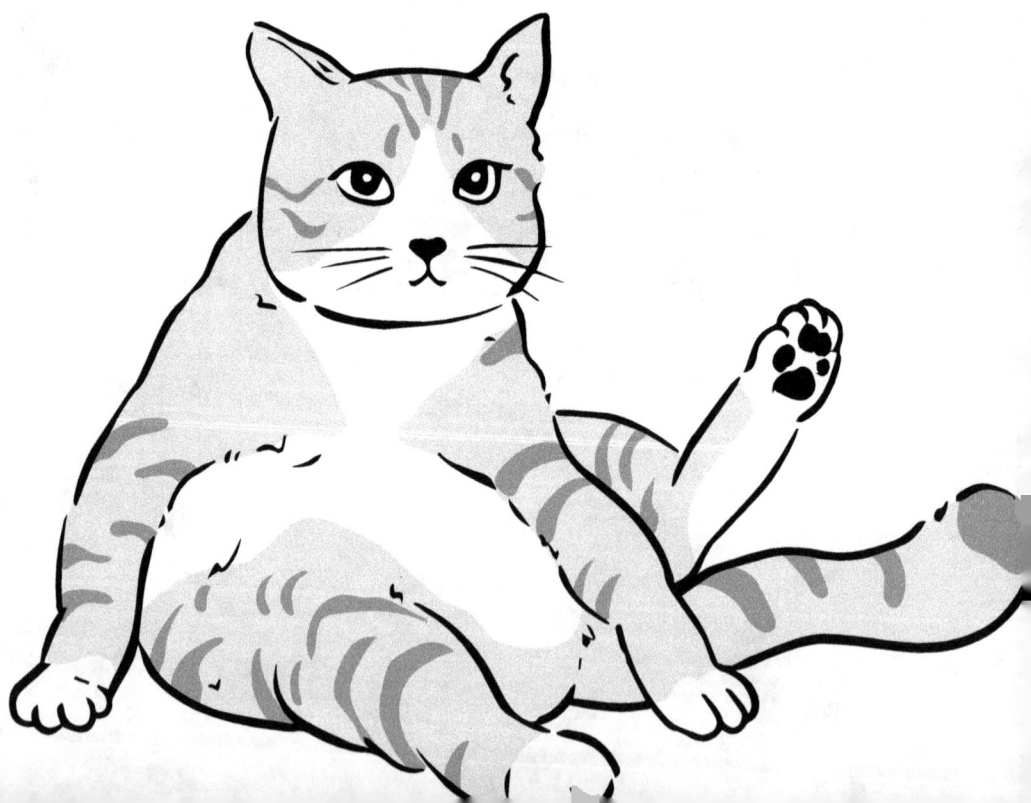

I am intelligent and wise, making smart decisions for myself.

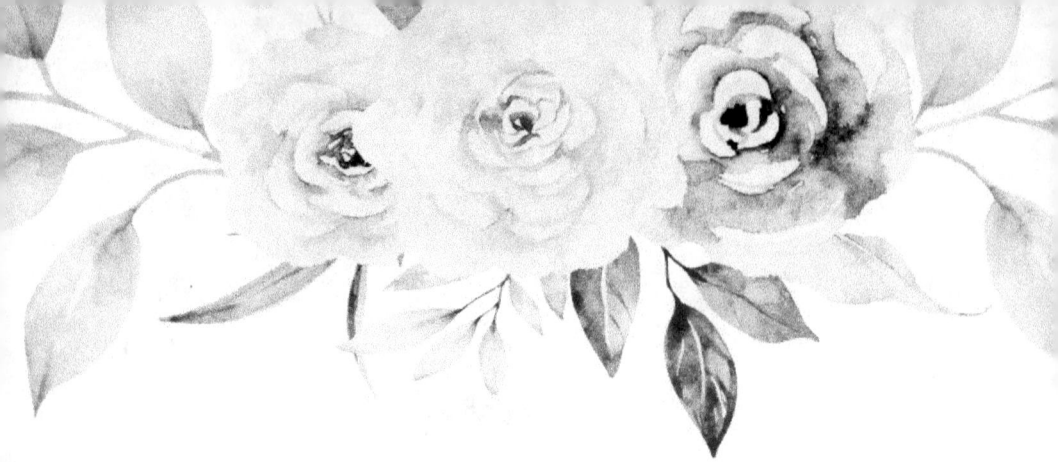

I attract abundance and prosperity into my life.

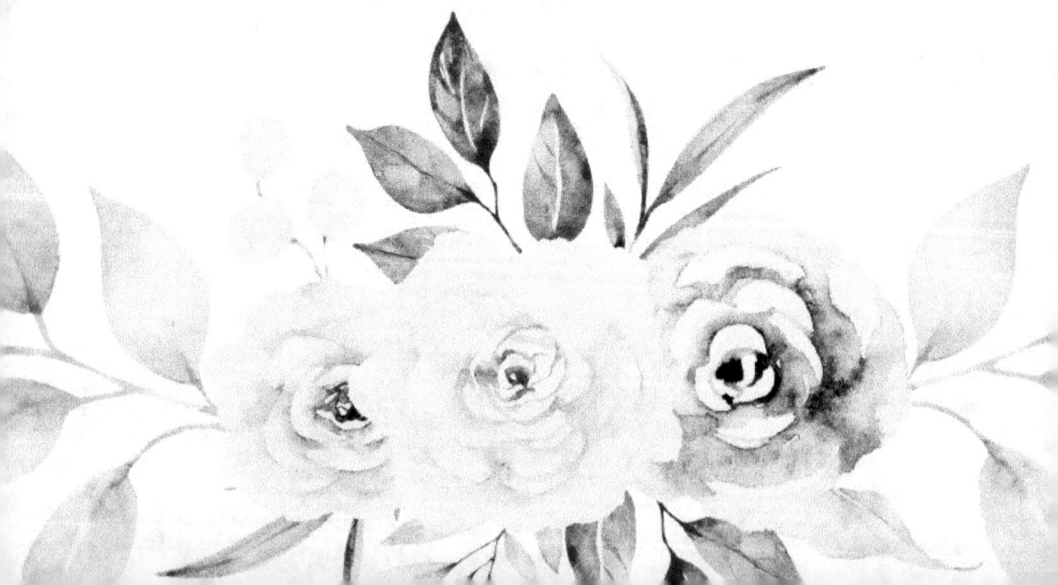

I am strong, resilient, and can handle anything that comes my way.

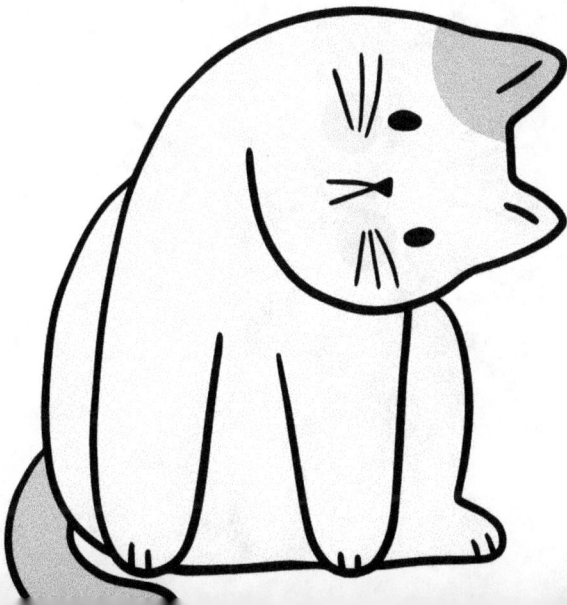

I embrace my uniqueness and celebrate my individuality.

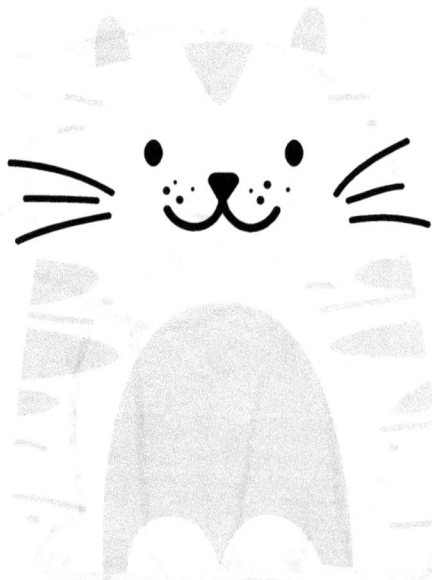

I am a
valuable
and
important
part of my
community.

I forgive myself for any past mistakes and embrace growth.

I set healthy boundaries that protect my well-being.

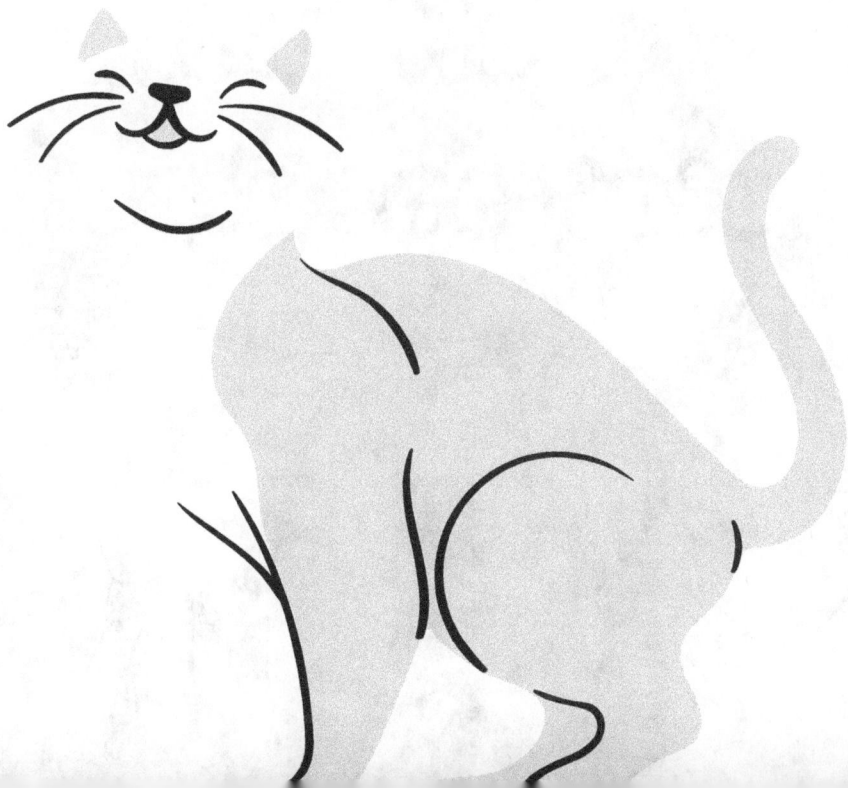

I am open to giving and receiving love in all my relationships.

I am
confident in
expressing
my thoughts
and feelings.

I am a kind and compassionate person, both to myself and others.

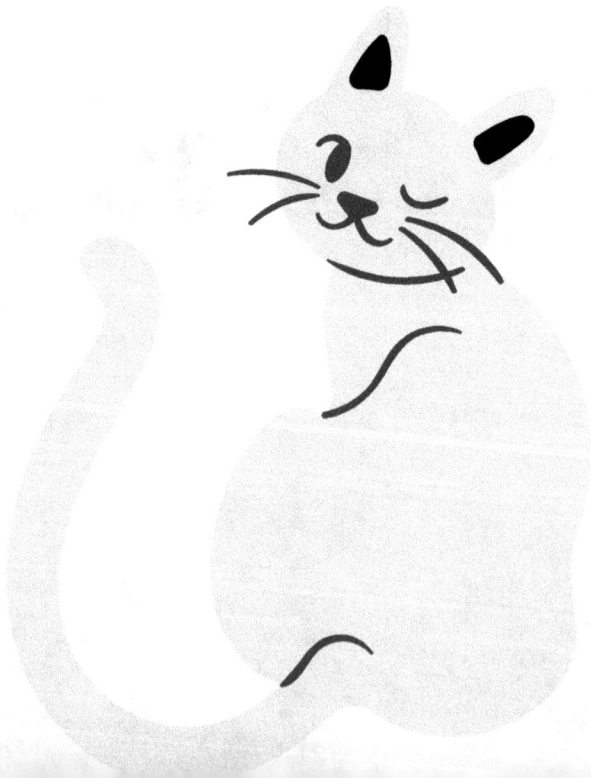

I trust my intuition and make decisions that align with my values.

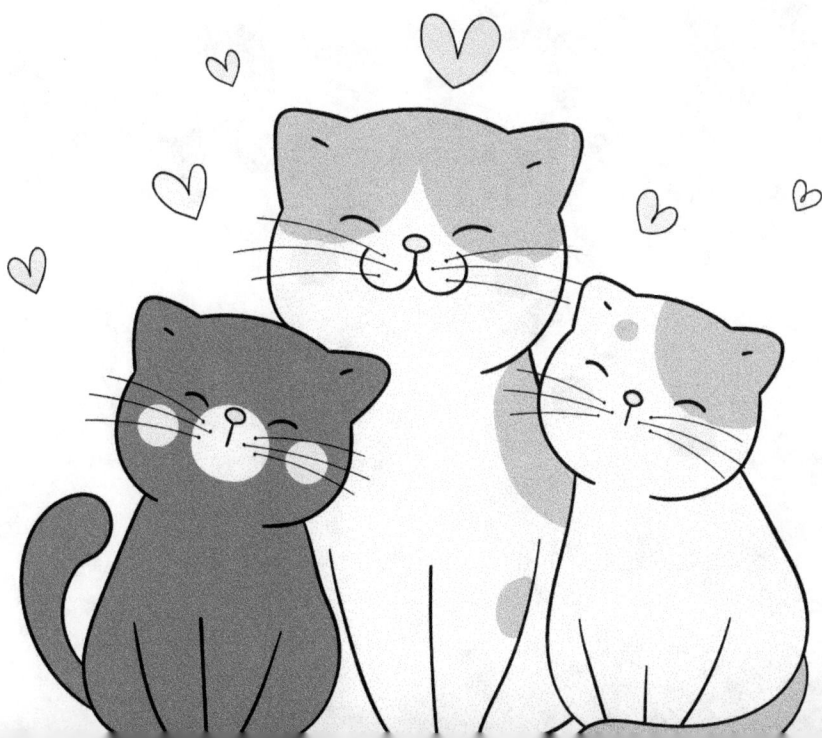

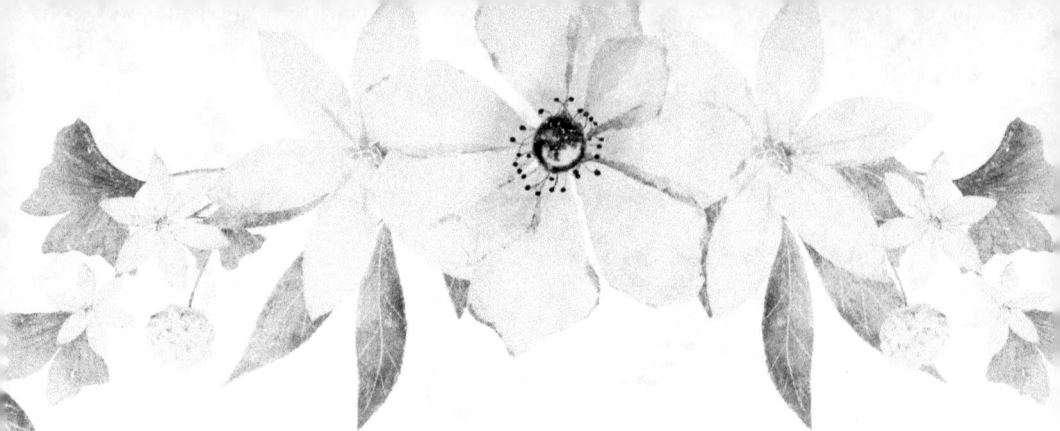

I am constantly growing and evolving into the best version of myself.

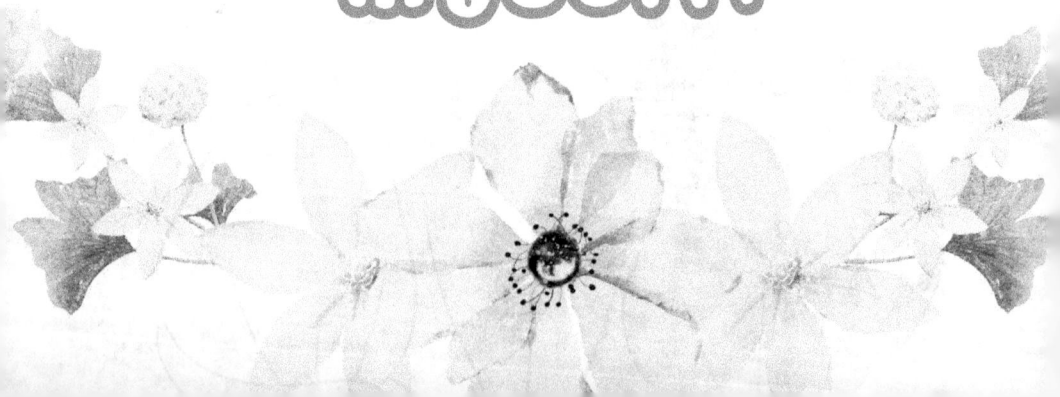

I am
deserving of
happiness and
fulfillment in
all aspects of
life.

I am deserving of success and recognition for my achievements.

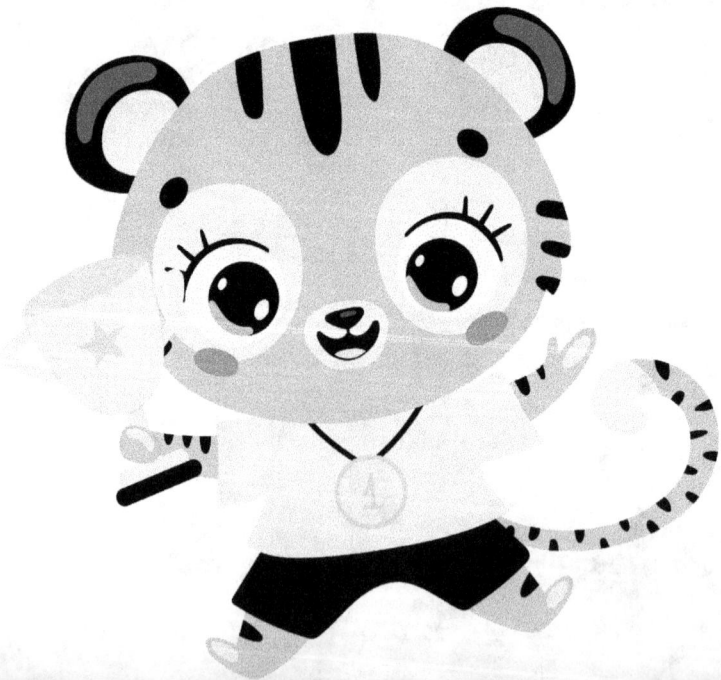

I am a leader, making positive impacts on those around me.

I am creative and capable of achieving my dreams.

I am in
control of
my thoughts
and
emotions.

I treat myself and others with respect and kindness.

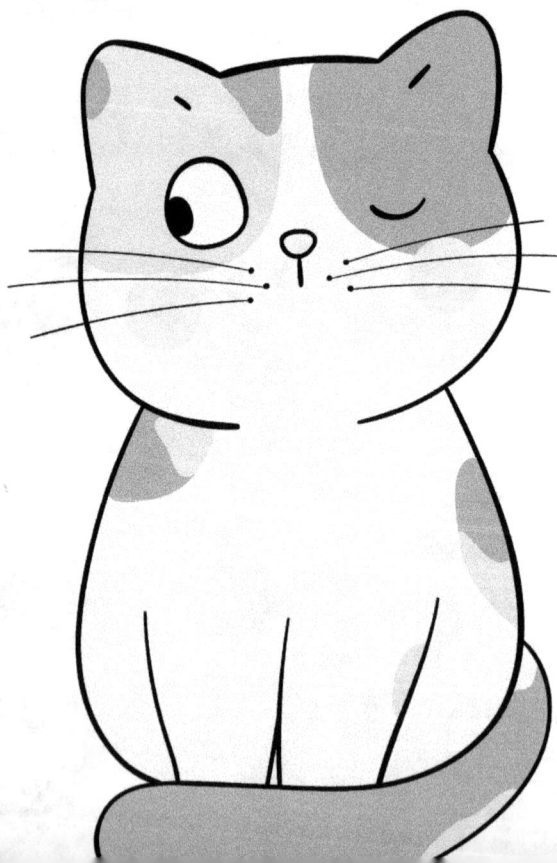

I am a source
of inspiration
and
empowerment
to those around
me.

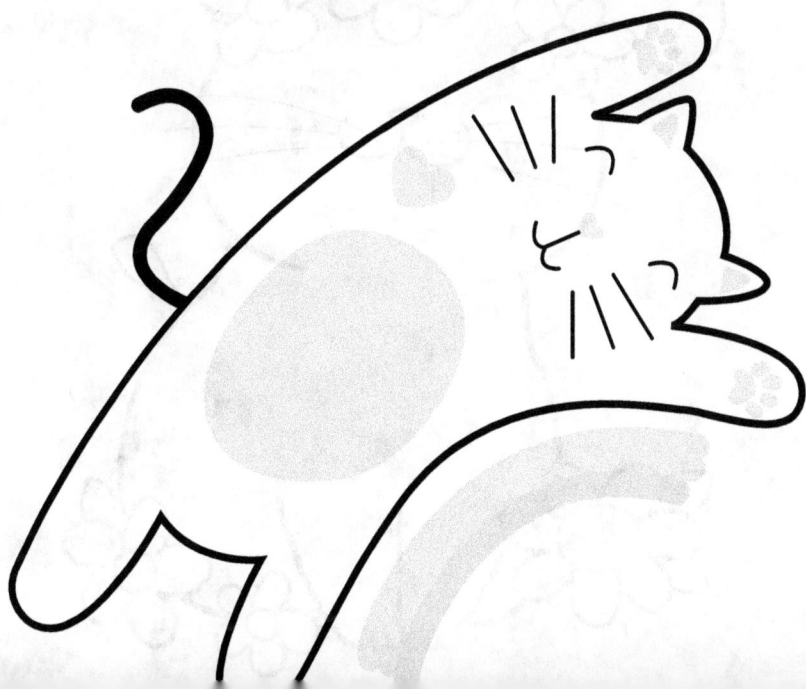

I trust in my abilities and make confident decisions.

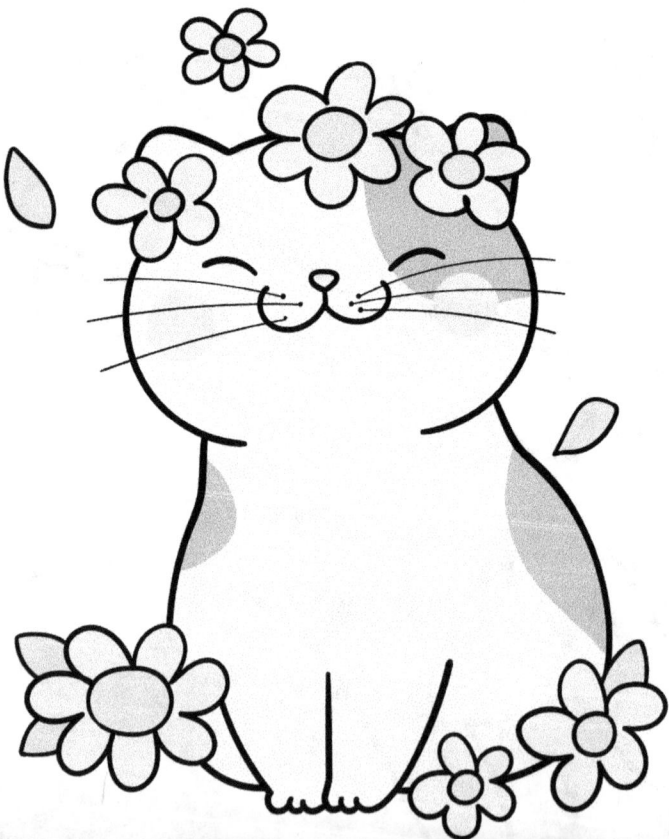

www.ingramcontent.com/pod-product-compliance
Lightning Source LLC
Chambersburg PA
CBHW060524280326
41933CB00014B/3096